The Medical SOCIAL WORKER PLAYBOOK:

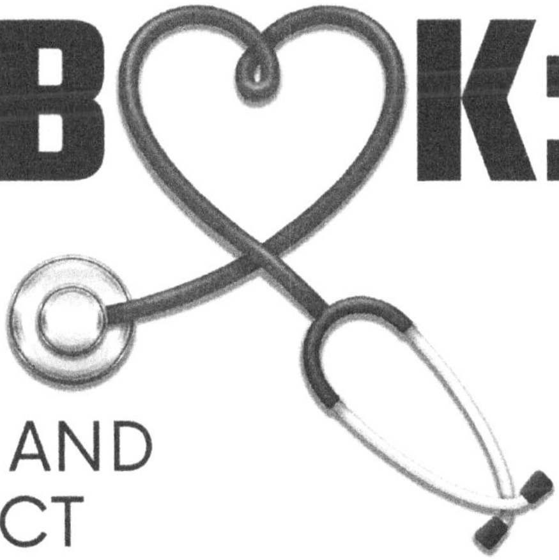

25 KEYS TO COMPETENCE, COMPASSION, AND CLINICAL IMPACT

DR. KENSHARA CRAVENS-KNOXSON
LMSW, LGSW,CCM, SAP, LCDC (CI)

Produced for Publication by The Author's Pen, LLC
PO Box 16314
Fort Worth, Texas 76132
www.tapwriting.com

The Medical Social Worker Playbook:
25 Keys to Competence, Compassion, and Clinical Impact

/Kenshara Cravens-Knoxson

-- 1st printed. ISBN 978-1-948248-66-2

Note: Portions of this book were developed with the assistance of ChatGPT, a language model created by OpenAI, to help organize ideas, generate drafts, and refine content. All content has been reviewed and edited for accuracy and relevance by the author.

OpenAI. (2024). ChatGPT (Mar 14 version) [Large language model]. https://chat.openai.com/

In-text: (OpenAI, 2024)

Acknowledgements

This book is the result of lived experience, long nights, full hearts, and the steady belief that social work, especially in healthcare, is both a calling and a craft.

To the patients and families who allowed me into some of the most intimate moments of their lives: thank you. Your resilience, vulnerability, and trust have shaped the deepest parts of my professional identity. I carry your stories with care.

To my colleagues, nurses, physicians, chaplains, therapists, case managers, and especially fellow social workers, your collaboration, wisdom, and humor have kept me grounded in the most complex of circumstances. You've reminded me that this work is never done alone.

To my mentors and supervisors, thank you for creating space for reflection, growth, and advocacy. You taught me that being ethical is more important than being easy and that being present is often more powerful than being right.

To the next generation of medical social workers, I wrote this for you. May this book serve as a guide, a mirror, and a reminder that what you do matters more than you may ever fully see.

Finally, to my family and loved ones, thank you for the patience, encouragement, and grace that allowed me to write through work, life, and everything in between. Your belief in me is woven into every page.

With deep gratitude.

Contents

Introduction

Medical social work is a field where knowledge, advocacy, and empathy intersect. It demands not only clinical expertise but also the ability to navigate complex healthcare systems, collaborate with multidisciplinary teams, and support patients and families through some of life's most challenging moments. Whether you're just starting your career or you're a seasoned professional, this book is designed to provide essential insights that every medical social worker should know.

Throughout my career, I've encountered the common struggles, unexpected challenges, and moments of profound fulfillment that define this work. I've also seen firsthand the gaps in formal education that leave many social workers feeling unprepared for the realities of medical settings. This book distills practical wisdom, real-world strategies, and key takeaways that will help you not only survive but thrive in this demanding profession.

From mastering hospital policies and understanding insurance systems to navigating ethical dilemmas and preventing burnout, these 25 lessons serve as a roadmap for success. Each chapter offers practical guidance, case examples, and actionable tips to help you confidently step into your role as a medical social worker.

No matter where you are in your journey, I hope this book serves as a valuable companion—one that empowers you to advocate effectively, maintain your well-being, and make a meaningful difference in the lives of those you serve.

Let's dive in.

The Heart of Patient and Family Care

Before you can effectively advocate, counsel, or coordinate care, you need a strong clinical foundation. In medical social work, clinical doesn't only mean diagnosing mental health conditions—it also means understanding the systems, language, and psychosocial impact of illness and treatment. This section lays the groundwork for everything that follows.

You'll explore how to:

- Speak the language of healthcare professionals
- Navigate complex systems and settings
- Understand common medical conditions
- Conduct comprehensive psychosocial assessments
- Practice trauma-informed care in every interaction

These skills will help you become a trusted member of the care team—someone who can communicate across disciplines, support patients through crisis, and bridge the gap between medicine and humanity.

CHAPTER 1:
Understanding Medical Terminology

In medical social work, language matters. A lot.

You're in the room with physicians, nurses, case managers, and therapists. You hear acronyms, abbreviations, and clinical language flying across the room. You're expected to keep up—and also to slow down and help the patient and their family understand what's going on.

No one expects you to be a medical expert, but you do need to be medically **fluent**. That fluency allows you to advocate effectively, participate confidently in interdisciplinary discussions, and earn the trust of both patients and colleagues.

If you're not familiar with the terms being used, you can miss critical details. You may overlook safety concerns during discharge planning, misinterpret treatment goals, or delay connecting a patient with the right level of care.

When you *are* fluent, you can translate complex information into compassionate, clear language that patients can understand and act on. That's powerful.

Real Talk: Why This Matters

Let's say a patient is being treated for "CHF exacerbation." A nurse asks you to help plan for discharge. If you don't know that CHF stands for **congestive heart failure**—and that "exacerbation" means it's getting worse—you may miss the urgency. You might underestimate how exhausted the patient feels, or the risk of returning home without proper support.

Or consider a patient who is "full code." Without knowing that this means the team will perform all life-saving interventions, you could have a very different conversation with the family than intended.

Language is a tool. When you use it well, it builds bridges. When you fumble it, it can widen gaps.

Common Medical Terms You Should Know

Term	What It Means
A&O x3 or x4	Alert and Oriented (to person, place, time, and sometimes situation)
ARDS	Acute Respiratory Distress Syndrome – a severe lung condition
BKA	Below Knee Amputation
CABG	Coronary Artery Bypass Graft – heart surgery
C. diff	Clostridioides difficile – a contagious bacterial infection in the gut
Dx	Diagnosis
DVT	Deep Vein Thrombosis – blood clot in a vein, often in the leg
Foley	A type of catheter inserted into the bladder
FTT	Failure to Thrive – often used for elderly or children with significant decline
G-tube	Gastrostomy tube – feeding tube inserted into the stomach

H&P	History and Physical – provider's initial assessment
H&P	History and Physical (provider's comprehensive exam and documentation)
I&O	Intake and Output – how much fluid a patient takes in and expels
Infarct	Tissue damage due to lack of blood flow (e.g., heart attack, stroke)
Ischemia	Inadequate blood supply to an organ or part of the body
LOC	Level of Consciousness
MRI	Magnetic Resonance Imaging – a diagnostic scan
NPO	Nothing by Mouth (patient cannot eat or drink)
PEG Tube	Percutaneous Endoscopic Gastrostomy – long-term feeding tube
PT/OT/ST	Physical, Occupational, and Speech Therapy
Psych Eval	Psychiatric Evaluation – mental health assessment
RRT	Rapid Response Team – summoned for acute patient deterioration
Sepsis	A serious, potentially life-threatening response to infection
SOB	Shortness of Breath
Stat	Immediately (from Latin *statim*)
Telemetry	Continuous heart monitoring unit

TIA	Transient Ischemic Attack – "mini-stroke" with no permanent damage
TPN	Total Parenteral Nutrition – IV nutrition for patients who can't eat
Vent	Ventilator – machine to support breathing
Wound Vac	A device to help wounds heal through suction
XR or X-ray	Radiographic imaging tool

You'll learn more terms on the job. What matters most is your willingness to ask, clarify, and grow.

Practical Tips

- **Make your own glossary** – Keep a notebook or digital list of unfamiliar terms you hear. Look them up after rounds.
- **Use plain language** – Practice translating terms into patient-friendly explanations. Say "serious infection" instead of "sepsis."
- **Ask for clarification** – Don't pretend to know what something means. Asking shows initiative, not ignorance.
- **Review documentation carefully** – Clinical notes are full of terms that can shape your intervention plan.

Try This: Conversation Practice

Next time you hear a term you're not familiar with, challenge yourself to do three things:

1. Write it down.
2. Look it up later.

3. Try explaining it to someone in everyday language.

   This practice will build both your confidence and your clinical voice.

Reflection Questions

- What medical terms have you heard but never fully understood?
- How has not knowing certain terms impacted your ability to support a patient?
- What steps can you take to become more confident in medical language?

CHAPTER 2:
Navigating Health Systems

Being a great medical social worker isn't just about what you *do*—it's also about what you *understand*. To be effective in your role, you need to understand the inner workings of the healthcare system you're operating within.

Hospitals and medical facilities are complex, hierarchical, fast-paced environments filled with rules, roles, and routines that aren't always obvious. If you don't understand how patients move through the system—or who holds which responsibilities—you can end up stuck, overwhelmed, or overlooked.

But when you *do* understand the system, you can cut through red tape, anticipate the next steps, and advocate with precision. You'll know who to talk to, when to escalate an issue, and how to keep patients from falling through the cracks.

Healthcare Settings You May Work In

As a medical social worker, you may work across a range of settings:

- **Acute Care Hospitals** – Fast-paced, short-term medical care, including ER and inpatient floors.
- **Long-Term Acute Care (LTAC)** – Extended hospitalization for medically complex patients.
- **Rehabilitation Facilities** – Short- or long-term recovery for injuries, strokes, or post-surgery.

- **Skilled Nursing Facilities (SNFs)** – Provide 24/7 nursing and rehabilitation services.
- **Outpatient Clinics** – Focused care for chronic conditions or specialty services.
- **Hospice or Home Health** – End-of-life care or medical services delivered in the home.

Each setting has different workflows, policies, and expectations—but your core skills stay the same.

The Interdisciplinary Team: Who's Who

Understanding team roles helps you know where you fit—and how you can help the team function better.

Role	**Primary Responsibilities**
Physician	Leads medical diagnosis and treatment decisions
Nurse	Coordinates clinical care, medications, and patient monitoring
Case Manager	Works with insurance, discharge planning, and logistics
Therapists (PT/OT/ST)	Assess mobility, functioning, and rehab needs
Pharmacist	Manages medication safety and interactions
Social Worker (You!)	Provides psychosocial assessment, crisis intervention, counseling, care coordination, and advocacy

When you understand what each person does, you can advocate more effectively—and avoid duplication or confusion.

Navigating Common Healthcare Processes

- **Rounds** – Daily team meetings to review patients' conditions and plans.
- **Utilization Review** – Determines if hospital stays and services are medically necessary.
- **Discharge Planning** – Begins on admission and involves coordinating the safest transition possible.
- **Referrals** – Connecting patients to post-acute services like home health, hospice, or community support.

If you know how these processes work, you'll be able to help patients move smoothly through the system and reduce delays.

Payor Sources Matter

Not everything is covered, and who's paying often dictates what options are available.

Payor Type	Key Points
Medicare	Federal insurance for people 65+ or with disabilities
Medicaid	State-funded insurance for low-income individuals
Private Insurance	Varies widely—know which services require authorization
Self-Pay/ Uninsured	Often requires creative problem-solving and charity programs

Understanding these basics can help you plan realistic discharges and set expectations for patients and families.

Real Talk: Systems Can Be Frustrating

Yes, the system is full of flaws. Bureaucracy, insurance limits, and institutional barriers are real. But knowing how to work *within* the system—even as you push for change—can be a powerful form of advocacy.

The more familiar you are with the rules, roles, and roadblocks, the more impact you can make on behalf of your patients.

Practical Tips

- **Know your key contacts** – Build relationships with discharge planners, community liaisons, and financial counselors.
- **Stay calm under pressure** – Hospitals run on urgency. Bring calm, clarity, and solutions.
- **Anticipate needs** – Don't wait until discharge day to start asking about support systems or housing.

Reflection Questions

- What healthcare settings have you worked in or observed?
- Where have you felt most confident—and most confused—navigating the system?
- How can you better understand the "flow" of your workplace?

CHAPTER 3:

Common Health Conditions and Comorbidities

Medical social workers work with people experiencing illness, injury, and chronic health conditions—and often, more than one at a time. While you're not a medical provider, having a working knowledge of **common diagnoses and comorbidities** helps you connect the dots between physical health and psychosocial needs.

Why does this matter? Because illness affects every part of a person's life—not just their body. Understanding what patients are facing medically allows you to ask better questions, anticipate complications, and coordinate the right support.

The Most Common Conditions You'll Encounter

Here's a look at common diagnoses in inpatient and outpatient healthcare settings, and how they might affect social work practice:

Condition	Psychosocial Considerations
Stroke	Sudden disability, speech loss, depression, family caregiver burden
Cancer	Fear of death, body image changes, financial strain, treatment access

Heart Failure (CHF)	Fatigue, mobility issues, frequent hospitalizations, end-of-life planning
Diabetes	Diet, medication access, financial cost, complications like vision loss or amputation
COPD	Shortness of breath, oxygen use, depression, home safety concerns
Dementia/ Alzheimer's	Safety, caregiver burnout, decision-making, long-term care planning
Substance Use Disorders	Risk of readmission, withdrawal concerns, need for treatment referrals
Mental Health Diagnoses (Depression, Anxiety, Bipolar)	Medication adherence, stigma, support systems, co-occurring issues
Chronic Pain	Functional limitations, opioid use, disability paperwork, isolation
End-Stage Renal Disease (ESRD)	Dialysis access, transportation, the emotional toll of chronic treatment

These are just a few—but even a basic awareness can make a big difference in how you support the person behind the diagnosis.

What Are Comorbidities?

Comorbidity refers to the presence of two or more conditions at the same time. For example:

- A patient with **diabetes and depression**
- An older adult with **dementia and congestive heart failure**
- A cancer survivor who also struggles with **substance use**

When conditions overlap, the complexity increases—not just medically, but socially and emotionally. Medication routines are harder to follow. Stress and hopelessness increase. Support systems wear thin.

Social workers are uniquely positioned to help patients *navigate these overlaps*—and to ensure the care plan reflects the full person, not just one diagnosis at a time.

How This Affects Discharge Planning and Advocacy

Knowing the likely progression of a condition helps you:

- Set realistic expectations for recovery
- Recommend the appropriate level of care (home health, SNF, hospice)
- Coordinate durable medical equipment (DME) or rehab services
- Prepare patients and families for what's next

For example, a patient with **advanced COPD** may need oxygen, pulmonary rehab, and conversations about future care wishes. A person with **dementia** may require 24/7 supervision and legal planning for medical power of attorney.

Practical Tips

- **Don't memorize everything**—focus on the conditions you see most often in your setting.
- **Ask the team**—nurses and doctors are often happy to explain a diagnosis in plain language.
- **Create a "cheat sheet"** for quick reference. Include signs/symptoms, typical challenges, and key community resources.

Reflection Questions

- What are the top 3 conditions you encounter most in your current role?
- What challenges do patients with those conditions often face?
- How can you improve your understanding of the medical and emotional impact of those diagnoses?

CHAPTER 4:
Conducting Psychosocial Assessments

In medical social work, the psychosocial assessment is your foundation. It's how you move from treating symptoms to supporting *people*. You are often the only one on the care team asking about a patient's life outside the hospital walls—housing, mental health, trauma history, support systems, safety, and dignity.

A good psychosocial assessment doesn't just fill out a form. It paints a picture of the person behind the diagnosis.

What Is a Psychosocial Assessment?

A psychosocial assessment is a clinical tool that gathers information about a patient's:

- Mental and emotional health
- Social supports and family dynamics
- Housing, income, employment, and education
- Substance use history
- Legal or safety concerns
- Cultural and spiritual beliefs
- Barriers to care (transportation, language, cognitive ability)

The goal is to understand the whole person so that interventions—whether discharge plans, therapy, or referrals—are effective.

Why It Matters in Medical Settings

Patients are often overwhelmed, scared, in pain, or experiencing trauma. You may only get a few minutes with them. But what you learn in those few minutes can change the entire trajectory of care.

For example:

- Discovering a patient lives alone on the third floor with no elevator may alter a discharge plan.
- Noticing signs of caregiver burnout may prompt a family meeting or respite referral.
- Uncovering a history of trauma may shape how you approach treatment planning.

Key Domains to Explore

Domain	What to Ask or Observe
Mental Health	Mood, orientation, history of diagnoses, psychiatric care
Substance Use	Current or past use, treatment history, impact on health
Support System	Who helps at home? Who visits? Any strained relationships?
Housing & Safety	Is the home safe and accessible? Risk of eviction or violence?
Income & Insurance	Employment status, disability benefits, financial strain
Spirituality	Beliefs that affect coping or treatment decisions
Legal Needs	POA, guardianship, custody, restraining orders

Cultural Factors	Language, decision-making norms, health beliefs

Practical Tips for a Strong Assessment

- **Ask open-ended questions.** ("Tell me about who helps you at home.")
- **Use warmth and curiosity.** People respond to nonjudgmental presence.
- **Normalize sensitive topics.** ("Many people find it hard to afford medications. How about you?")
- **Be culturally responsive.** Don't assume what's "normal" for you is true for everyone.
- **Document what matters.** Write clinically relevant notes but with compassion and precision.

The Art of Building Rapport Quickly

You often don't have time to "build a relationship" in the traditional sense. But you *can* build rapport in the first 60 seconds by:

- Introducing yourself clearly
- Explaining your role and how you can help
- Asking permission to talk and listening actively

That human connection opens the door for deeper, more honest assessments.

Reflection Questions

- What part of the psychosocial assessment do you feel most confident in?
- What domains do you tend to rush or overlook?
- How do you adjust your approach for different patient populations?

CHAPTER 5:
Practicing Trauma-Informed Care

Every patient brings more than a medical chart into the room—they bring a story. Many of those stories include trauma: childhood abuse, systemic oppression, medical mistreatment, community violence, or simply the trauma of being sick and vulnerable in a healthcare setting.

As a medical social worker, your job is to create a sense of safety, dignity, and empowerment—even when everything else feels out of control. That's what trauma-informed care is all about.

What Is Trauma-Informed Care?

Trauma-informed care is not a technique—it's a mindset. It's the intentional practice of recognizing the presence and impact of trauma in patients' lives and adapting your approach to avoid re-traumatization.

According to the Substance Abuse and Mental Health Services Administration (SAMHSA), trauma-informed care is based on **six key principles**:

1. **Safety**
2. **Trustworthiness and Transparency**
3. **Peer Support**
4. **Collaboration and Mutuality**
5. **Empowerment, Voice, and Choice**
6. **Cultural, Historical, and Gender Considerations**

You don't have to know a person's trauma history to offer trauma-informed care. You just have to assume that *someone in every room has one*—and act accordingly.

Why It Matters in Medical Social Work

Hospitals and medical systems can be triggering for trauma survivors:

- Lack of privacy
- Power differentials
- Invasive procedures
- Fast-paced, impersonal communication
- Historical mistrust of medical institutions (especially among marginalized communities)

Trauma-informed social workers slow things down, explain what's happening, offer choices, and center the patient's sense of control—because control is often the first thing trauma takes away.

What Trauma Can Look Like in Healthcare

Signs	Examples
Hypervigilance	Patient is tense, constantly watching the door, afraid of being touched
Shutdown or Dissociation	Patient becomes silent, avoids eye contact, appears "checked out"
Anger or Defensiveness	Resistance to treatment or care team, especially if not feeling heard
Distrust	Refusal to sign paperwork, fear of being lied to, hesitation to disclose history

These reactions aren't personal—they're protective. Your job is to respond, not react.

Practical Trauma-Informed Strategies

- **Always introduce yourself.** Explain your role and why you're there.
- **Ask for permission.** "Is it okay if we talk for a few minutes now?"
- **Use plain language.** Avoid jargon and acronyms.
- **Offer choices.** Even small ones help restore agency ("Would you like to talk here or in the family room?").
- **Validate their experience.** "That sounds really overwhelming. You're doing the best you can."
- **Be aware of your tone and body language.** A calm, open, non-threatening presence matters.

Being Trauma-Informed with Staff, Too

It's not just patients—colleagues carry trauma too. Nurses, techs, and even physicians experience secondary trauma, burnout, and moral injury. You can model trauma-informed care in how you treat *everyone*.

Reflection Questions

- How do you recognize trauma responses in patients or families?
- What strategies have helped you de-escalate tense or emotional moments?
- What parts of your practice still need to be more trauma-informed?

Supporting Patients and Families

In Section 2, you explored the emotional heart of medical social work—your role as a steady, skilled presence during some of the most vulnerable moments in a person's life.

Each chapter emphasized a different layer of support, from crisis stabilization to discharge planning, and from honoring grief to respecting cultural values. Together, they form a toolkit for compassionate, responsive care.

Key Takeaways:

- **Crisis intervention** requires clarity, calm, and empathy. You are often the first support in a moment of shock or fear.
- **Grief and loss** deserve space, not solutions. You don't fix grief—you witness it, validate it, and hold space for healing.
- **Cultural humility** is a mindset, not a skill. Ask, listen, and adapt your care to meet patients where they are.
- **Discharge planning** starts early and depends on your ability to coordinate resources, anticipate needs, and communicate effectively.
- **Advance care planning** is about dignity, choice, and preparation. You help patients and families make informed decisions, even when it's hard.

Guiding Principles:

- **Be human first.** The best clinical skill is often presence.
- **Practice cultural responsiveness.** Every family, belief system, and expression of distress deserves respect.
- **Empower the patient's voice.** Even in medical systems built on authority, you can center the patient's autonomy.
- **Know your resources.** Having the right contact at the right time can change everything.
- **Debrief and reflect often.** Supporting others through pain and uncertainty takes a toll. Make space to process your own emotional responses.

This section reminded you that while policies, diagnoses, and treatment plans are part of the job, the *people* are the reason you do it.

CHAPTER 6:
Crisis Intervention in Medical Settings

In medical social work, a crisis can occur at any moment. A sudden death. A life-changing diagnosis. A traumatic injury. A child in distress. A family in conflict. When a crisis hits, **you** are often the one called to respond.

You don't have the luxury of preparation or perfect timing. Crisis intervention in healthcare requires calm, confidence, and clarity—even when you're walking into the unknown.

But it's also one of the most meaningful parts of the work. You get to be the steady hand, the clear voice, and the compassionate witness when someone's world has just shifted.

What Is Crisis?

A crisis is not just an event—it's a person's perception that what is happening exceeds their current ability to cope. In healthcare, crises often involve:

- A sudden loss or unexpected bad news
- A traumatic or disfiguring event
- Fear for one's life or a loved one's
- A mental health emergency
- Disrupted caregiving plans

- Emotional overwhelm triggered by hospitalization

When you understand what crisis feels like—not just what it looks like—you can respond more skillfully.

The Role of the Social Worker in Crisis

As a medical social worker in a crisis, your role is to:

- **De-escalate emotions** (fear, anger, panic, grief)
- **Provide grounding and clarity**
- **Mobilize support** (family, clergy, care team)
- **Protect safety** (assess for harm to self/others)
- **Support decision-making** (especially under emotional duress)
- **Advocate for the patient/family** during team discussions

You may not be able to change the outcome—but you can change how the moment is experienced.

Steps for Effective Crisis Intervention (The "ABCDE" Approach)

Step	What to Do
A – Assess	Evaluate safety, mental status, coping, and needs
B – Build Rapport	Use warmth, presence, and nonjudgmental tone
C – Contain Emotions	Normalize reactions; give space to express feelings
D – Develop a Plan	Clarify options, next steps, or available supports

E – Engage Resources	Involve family, spiritual care, psych, or other supports

This approach helps you stay structured even when everything feels chaotic.

Crisis Scenarios You May Encounter

- Family breakdown after a patient's terminal prognosis
- Suicide attempt or disclosure of suicidal ideation
- Parents grieving the loss of a newborn in the NICU
- A patient refusing life-saving treatment due to fear
- Violent trauma or mass casualty situations
- Domestic violence disclosures during hospitalization

Each requires sensitivity, systems knowledge, and self-awareness.

What NOT to Do in a Crisis

- Don't minimize. ("At least they lived.")
- Don't jump to solutions. Sometimes holding space is the solution.
- Don't impose your own beliefs. Honor what matters to *them*.
- Don't go in alone if the situation feels unsafe—bring backup.

Self-Regulation for the Social Worker

Crisis intervention takes energy. To stay grounded:

- Breathe slowly and deeply.
- Notice your own emotional reactions and center yourself.
- Debrief with trusted colleagues when needed.
- Practice nonattachment—be present, but don't carry it all home.

Reflection Questions

- What's the most challenging crisis you've responded to?
- What did you do well? What would you do differently next time?
- What helps you stay grounded and present in emotionally intense situations?

CHAPTER 7:
Grief, Loss, and End-of-Life Support

Grief walks into the room long before a patient dies. It shows up in quiet moments, loud arguments, silent tears, and decisions no one wants to make. As a medical social worker, you don't just encounter death—you walk alongside people *through it.*

You don't need the perfect words. You need presence, permission, and patience. This chapter will help you support patients and families through end-of-life and loss in a way that honors their humanity and yours.

Understanding Grief in Medical Settings

Grief in healthcare isn't always linear or obvious. It might look like:

- Anger at the staff or system
- Denial of the prognosis
- Guilt about decisions made (or not made)
- Hopelessness or spiritual questioning
- Withdrawal, silence, or refusal to engage

Grief isn't just about death. People grieve the loss of independence, function, certainty, roles, and identity. Your job is to recognize those losses, even when others don't name them.

Your Role at End-of-Life

As a social worker, you bring calm to chaos, compassion to confusion, and clarity to hard choices. You may be asked to:

- Facilitate goals-of-care conversations
- Coordinate hospice referrals
- Help complete advance directives
- Provide anticipatory grief support
- Mediate family conflicts
- Advocate for patient dignity and comfort

Sometimes, the most powerful thing you can do is sit in silence and *be there*.

What to Say When Words Are Hard

Instead of...	Try...
"They're in a better place."	"This is incredibly hard. I'm here with you."
"Everything happens for a reason."	"What you're feeling makes total sense."
"At least..."	*Avoid comparisons or minimizing. Stay present.*
"Let me know if you need anything."	"Would it help if I sat with you for a while?"

Cultural and Spiritual Sensitivity in Grief

Grief is shaped by culture, faith, family structure, and beliefs about death. Ask open-ended questions:

- "Are there any traditions or rituals that are important to you right now?"
- "How do you and your family usually cope with difficult times?"
- "Is there anyone you'd like me to call for support—spiritual, family, or otherwise?"

Don't assume that silence means peace or that tears mean crisis. Honor how people grieve—even if it looks different from your own.

Caring for Yourself When Facing Death

Bearing witness to death—especially repeatedly—is emotionally heavy. Build your own rituals for decompression:

- Take five minutes outside after a death
- Write a brief reflection
- Debrief with a colleague
- Use art, journaling, or grounding practices

Grief doesn't just affect patients and families. It lives in us, too, and must be tended with care.

Reflection Questions

- How has working with death shaped your personal views on life?
- What's one moment of presence you're proud of during a loss?
- How do you process your emotional responses to grief and death?

CHAPTER 8:
Practicing Cultural Competence in Healthcare

Culture is not just race or religion—it's language, identity, family structure, food, customs, worldview, and how people make meaning. In medical social work, cultural competence isn't optional. It's an ethical obligation and a professional necessity.

When you walk into a hospital room, you may encounter beliefs, norms, or expectations that differ from your own. Your role is to lead with humility—not to be the expert, but to be the learner.

What Cultural Competence Really Means

Cultural competence is the ability to understand, respect, and respond to people from diverse cultural backgrounds in ways that affirm their identity and support their care.

But more than competence, we're called to **cultural humility**: a lifelong commitment to self-reflection, checking power dynamics, and being open to correction.

What Culture Affects in Healthcare

Culture can influence:

- Beliefs about illness, healing, and medication
- Preferences for gender-specific providers

- Communication norms (direct vs. indirect)
- Role of family in decision-making
- Expressions of pain or grief
- Willingness to disclose personal information
- Understanding of mental health and disability
- Trust or distrust in medical institutions

Recognizing these factors helps prevent assumptions—and ensures care plans align with what the patient values.

Questions to Ask with Cultural Humility

- "What matters most to you as we plan your care?"
- "Are there any customs, practices, or beliefs we should be aware of?"
- "Who usually helps make medical decisions in your family?"
- "Are there any concerns you have about how your values are being respected here?"

You don't need to know every tradition—but you do need to ask the right questions.

Use of Language Services

Never rely on a family member, child, or staff person "who speaks a little Spanish" to interpret. **Always use professional interpreters** for medical conversations.

- Know how to request in-person, phone, or video interpreters
- Give patients extra time to process translated information
- Speak directly to the patient—not the interpreter
- Avoid using medical jargon that doesn't translate easily

Language access is a right—not a favor.

What Cultural Competence Looks Like in Practice

Scenario	Culturally Responsive Response
A patient declines hospice because "it means giving up."	Ask what "giving up" means to them. Explore goals of care using their language.
A family insists on aggressive treatment despite a poor prognosis.	Explore cultural or faith-based views on death, suffering, and miracles.
A patient is uncomfortable with a male provider.	Ask about preferences and advocate for alternatives when possible.
A patient uses traditional healing alongside Western medicine.	Avoid judgment. Ask how both approaches can be respected.

Avoiding Cultural Pitfalls

- Don't assume shared identity = shared beliefs.
- Don't pathologize cultural differences.
- Don't dismiss "noncompliance" without understanding barriers.
- Don't speak for communities you don't belong to—amplify voices instead.

Reflection Questions

- When have you been challenged by cultural differences in a patient interaction?
- What helped you connect—or what created distance?
- What are you doing to expand your cultural awareness?

CHAPTER 9:
Mastering Discharge Planning

In medical social work, discharge planning is where clinical insight meets logistical hustle. You are the bridge between the hospital and the next step—whether that's home, rehab, a shelter, or long-term care.

A strong discharge plan doesn't just meet the medical team's goals—it protects patient dignity, prevents readmission, and supports recovery.

What Discharge Planning Really Involves

Discharge planning is more than checking boxes on a form. It's a complex, collaborative process that includes:

- **Assessing needs:** What is the patient's physical, emotional, and social functioning?
- **Coordinating services:** Who's providing what? PT, home health, DME, medication delivery?
- **Addressing barriers:** Does the patient have a safe home? Transportation? Insurance coverage?
- **Educating and empowering:** Does the patient understand the plan? Are caregivers ready?

You're not just planning an exit—you're planning a safe transition.

Discharge Planning Starts on Admission

The best discharge plans are proactive, not reactive. Start asking early:

- Who will help you at home?
- What kind of home environment do you have?
- Have you needed services like home health or rehab before?
- Do you have transportation for follow-up appointments?

These questions open the door to early interventions—before discharge becomes a scramble.

Levels of Post-Acute Care: Know the Differences

Setting	Who It's For
Home with Home Health	Needs intermittent nursing or therapy but is homebound
Inpatient Rehab (IRF)	Must tolerate 3 hours/day of therapy, often after stroke/surgery
Skilled Nursing Facility (SNF)	Needs 24-hour nursing and rehab but not acute care
Long-Term Acute Care (LTAC)	Medically complex patients needing extended hospitalization
Hospice	Terminal illness with a life expectancy under 6 months
Shelter or Housing Referral	For patients experiencing homelessness or unsafe housing

Understanding these levels helps you set realistic expectations for patients and advocate effectively with the team.

Common Barriers to Safe Discharge

- Homelessness or housing instability
- Lack of caregivers or overwhelmed families

- Insurance denials or lack of coverage
- Behavioral health needs
- Substance use or cognitive impairment
- Transportation issues

You won't always have perfect solutions; your role is to identify the risks, explore resources, and document everything.

Keys to a Successful Discharge Plan

- **Start early.** Don't wait until discharge day.
- **Loop in the right people.** Include caregivers, therapists, and community providers.
- **Clarify the plan.** Patients often leave confused—simplify instructions.
- **Prepare for what could go wrong.** Missed meds? No rides? You'll need a backup plan.
- **Document clearly.** Note barriers, discussions, referrals, and decisions.

Discharge Isn't Just a Task—It's a Social Justice Issue

People with fewer resources are more likely to face unsafe discharges. Your role is to name those inequities and push for better options when possible. Advocate for patients who don't have the power to advocate for themselves.

Reflection Questions

- What makes a discharge plan "successful" in your eyes?
- How do you manage your role when the system offers limited or inequitable options?
- What tools or contacts do you rely on most during discharge planning?

CHAPTER 10:
Educating About Advance Directives

Talking about death is hard—but avoiding it doesn't make it go away. One of the most powerful roles a medical social worker plays is helping patients and families **make clear, informed choices** about care, especially before a crisis happens.

Advance care planning is about more than paperwork. It's about dignity, autonomy, and preparing for the unknown with clarity and compassion.

What Are Advance Directives?

Advance directives are legal documents that allow individuals to express their medical preferences **in case they become unable to speak for themselves**. These typically include:

Document	Purpose
Medical Power of Attorney (MPOA)	Appoints someone to make medical decisions if the patient can't
Living Will	States preferences for end-of-life care (e.g., feeding tubes, resuscitation)
Out-of-Hospital DNR	Indicates the patient does not want CPR outside the hospital setting

POLST/MOST Form	Provider Orders for Life-Sustaining Treatment – medical orders for seriously ill individuals

Each state has its own requirements, so be sure to use the correct forms and follow facility policy.

Why These Conversations Matter

When patients and families **don't** talk about care preferences, decisions get made in a vacuum—often during moments of fear and urgency. Families may feel guilt. Providers may offer aggressive treatment that doesn't align with the patient's values.

But when conversations happen early and often:

- Patients feel more in control
- Families feel less burdened
- Providers can deliver care aligned with the person's goals

Your role is to make space for those conversations—and provide tools that support them.

How to Start the Conversation

Instead of...	**Try...**
"Do you have a living will?"	"Have you had a chance to think about what kind of care you'd want if you couldn't speak for yourself?"
"You need to fill this out."	"This is a way to make sure your wishes are respected, no matter what happens."
"Who's in charge?"	"Is there someone you trust to make medical decisions for you if you can't?"

What Gets in the Way?

- **Fear of talking about death**
- **Family conflict or disagreement**
- **Cultural/religious views about end-of-life care**
- **Lack of understanding of medical terms**
- **The assumption that "they already know what I want"**

Your job isn't to push—but to create a space where questions are welcomed, and choices are honored.

Practical Tips for Social Workers

- **Know your state's forms.** Have copies ready, and know how to explain them simply.
- **Use real-life examples.** "Some people want everything done, some people don't. Where do you fall?"
- **Normalize the conversation.** Frame it as part of quality care—not a sign something bad is about to happen.
- **Loop in providers.** Collaborate with physicians and nurses to align messaging and clarify prognosis if needed.
- **Document the discussion.** Even if a form isn't completed, note preferences and family conversations.

Reflection Questions

- What's your comfort level in discussing advance directives?
- How have cultural or generational beliefs shaped these conversations in your work?
- What would you want if you were the patient—and how would you want someone to ask?

Ethics and Advocacy

In the fast-paced world of healthcare, decisions are made quickly, often under pressure. It's easy to lose sight of the human, the nuanced, and the ethical. But that's exactly where medical social workers thrive.

Section 3 centers on your role as a **protector of patient rights**, a **keeper of ethics**, and a **relentless advocate** for equity and access. When no one else in the room sees the risk, the injustice, or the deeper meaning—*you do*.

This section gives you tools to:

- Navigate ethical dilemmas with confidence and clarity
- Advocate for patient autonomy—even when others push back
- Understand mandated reporting requirements
- Promote health equity and call out systemic barriers
- Stay grounded in your values while operating in a complex medical system

You are the **moral anchor** in many rooms. This section affirms that role and helps you strengthen it, even in environments where ethics may take a backseat to efficiency.

CHAPTER 11:
Protecting Patient Rights

In healthcare, treatment can move fast—sometimes too fast. A plan gets made, a form is signed, and a procedure is scheduled. But lost in that speed is something sacred: the patient's **right to choose**.

As a medical social worker, one of your core responsibilities is to **protect autonomy**—to make sure patients understand what's happening, what their options are, and what they want. And when their voices are dismissed, it's your job to raise yours.

What Is Patient Autonomy?

Autonomy means the right to make decisions about one's own body and healthcare—even if others disagree.

It includes the right to:

- Be fully informed before consenting to care
- Refuse treatment (even if it's life-saving)
- Change their mind
- Appoint someone else to make decisions
- Ask questions without fear or pressure

Autonomy is not just a concept—it's an act of dignity.

What Informed Consent Really Means

True **informed consent** means the patient:

1. Receives accurate and complete information
2. Understands the risks, benefits, and alternatives
3. Has the capacity to make a decision
4. Makes the choice voluntarily, without coercion

If any one of these is missing, consent isn't fully informed—and you have an ethical obligation to speak up.

Common Situations Where Autonomy Is at Risk

- Family overrides the patient's wishes
- A patient agrees to a procedure out of fear, not understanding
- A nonverbal or cognitively impaired patient is assumed to be incapable
- Consent is obtained too quickly—or not at all
- Providers pressure patients into treatment based on their own values

In these moments, your presence matters. You are there to **slow things down** and center the person.

Assessing Capacity vs. Competency

- **Capacity** is a clinical judgment: Can the patient understand, evaluate, and express a decision?
- **Competency** is a legal determination made by a court.

If you suspect a patient lacks decision-making capacity, you may need to:

- Alert the medical team
- Request a capacity evaluation
- Identify legal surrogates (MPOA, next of kin)
- Review existing advance directives

Never assume based on age, disability, or diagnosis. Always assess.

Practical Advocacy Strategies

- **Clarify:** "Can you tell me in your own words what the plan is?"
- **Pause:** "Would you like more time to think about this before deciding?"
- **Reframe:** "There's no right or wrong decision—only what's right for you."
- **Document:** Note if the patient seemed confused, distressed, or unsure.
- **Escalate:** If you believe consent is invalid or autonomy is being violated, involve your ethics committee, supervisor, or patient advocacy department.

When Autonomy Conflicts with Family or Staff

It's not uncommon for families to say, "Just do whatever it takes," even when the patient has said otherwise. Or for a provider to push for aggressive treatment when a patient prefers comfort.

In these cases:

- Center the patient's stated values and wishes
- Facilitate family meetings to explore conflict
- Remind the team of ethical standards and patient rights
- Use phrases like, "What would this patient want if they could speak for themselves right now?"

Reflection Questions

- Have you ever seen a patient's autonomy disregarded? What did you do?
- What language helps you empower patients to speak up?
- How can you strengthen your role as an ethical advocate in your setting?

CHAPTER 12:
Mandated Reporting in Healthcare

As a medical social worker, you are not just a support person—you are also a **legally mandated reporter**. This means if you suspect abuse, neglect, or exploitation, you are required by law to report it.

This can be one of the most emotionally complex parts of your job. You may fear damaging trust, upsetting families, or creating unintended consequences. But your legal and ethical obligation is clear: **the safety of vulnerable people comes first**.

Who Are Mandated Reporters?

In most states, healthcare providers—including social workers, nurses, physicians, and therapists—are required to report suspected:

- Child abuse or neglect
- Abuse, neglect, or exploitation of older adults
- Abuse of adults with disabilities
- Human trafficking or sexual exploitation
- Domestic violence (in some states and under specific conditions)

You don't need proof. You don't need to be 100% certain. You only need **reasonable suspicion**.

What Counts as Reasonable Suspicion?

Signs in Children	Signs in Adults
Unexplained injuries or bruising	Poor hygiene or pressure sores
Fear of caregivers or flinching	Reports of verbal or physical abuse
Delays in seeking care	Confusion about finances or sudden changes in will
Inappropriate sexual knowledge	Isolation, intimidation, or fearfulness
Malnourishment or dehydration	Caregiver refuses to leave the room or answer questions

Listen to your gut. If something feels wrong—**report it**.

The Reporting Process

Each state has its own reporting process. Generally, it includes:

1. **Filing a report with the proper agency** (CPS, APS, law enforcement)
2. **Documenting the suspicion and your actions**
3. **Following your facility's internal protocols** (often informing risk management or a supervisor)

You can (and should) consult with a supervisor or legal/risk department—but **you cannot delegate the legal obligation to report**.

What to Say to Patients or Families

If possible and safe to do so, tell the patient or caregiver what's happening. Use calm, non-blaming language:

- "Because of what you shared, I'm required to make a report to help ensure everyone is safe."
- "My role is to connect people to help—not to get anyone in trouble."
- "I want you to have support, not shame."

Sometimes you won't be able to share—like in suspected child abuse or domestic violence where informing could escalate risk. Use professional judgment and follow policy.

Mandatory Doesn't Mean Mechanic

Reporting is about protection—not punishment. But it also comes with emotional weight:

- You may worry you're making a mistake.
- You may fear damaging your relationship with the patient.
- You may carry guilt or uncertainty about outcomes.

That's normal. Debrief with colleagues. Journal. Supervise. You're human, too.

Reflection Questions

- What's your process when you suspect abuse or neglect?
- How do you balance empathy with your legal responsibility?
- What do you need to feel more confident in your role as a mandated reporter?

CHAPTER 13:
Ethical Decision-Making in Complex Cases

Medical social work is full of gray areas. You'll find yourself in the middle of family conflicts, clashing professional opinions, cultural tensions, and emotionally charged decisions. Sometimes, there's no clear right answer—just the best decision based on the information you have, your ethical code, and the patient's values.

This is where social work ethics come alive—not in theory but as real-time guidance.

Common Ethical Dilemmas in Medical Settings

- A patient wants to leave AMA (Against Medical Advice), but the family insists they stay
- The team wants aggressive treatment; the patient wants comfort care
- A patient lacks capacity, and their surrogate makes decisions that conflict with prior wishes
- A minor discloses confidential information, but their parent demands details
- Staff treat certain patients dismissively due to behavioral or substance use issues

These situations can be morally distressing—and incredibly isolating if you're the only one speaking up.

Your Ethical Compass: NASW Code of Ethics

The **NASW Code of Ethics** is your professional guide. Key principles that apply in healthcare include:

Ethical Principle	Application
Dignity and Worth of the Person	Respect every patient's voice—even when it's inconvenient
Importance of Human Relationships	Mediate family conflict and promote communication
Integrity	Be honest with patients and team members, even when it's uncomfortable
Competence	Seek supervision when you're unsure or overwhelmed
Social Justice	Call out bias, inequity, and mistreatment when you see it

Ethics aren't just about doing what's legal—they're about doing what's *right*.

Using an Ethical Decision-Making Model

When you're stuck in a tough situation, walk through these steps:

1. **Identify the dilemma** – What values conflict?
2. **Consult policies and the Code of Ethics** – Are there clear standards or laws?
3. **Explore your emotional response** – Are your own beliefs influencing your reaction?
4. **Consult colleagues, ethics committees, or legal/risk teams** – Don't carry it alone.
5. **Evaluate the potential consequences** – Who is helped? Who is harmed?

6. **Document your process** – Show that your actions were thoughtful and ethically grounded.

When You're the Lone Voice in the Room

Sometimes, no one else sees the ethical issue but you. That doesn't mean you're wrong. It means your role is working.

Speak up respectfully:

- "I just want to pause for a second and make sure we're considering the patient's previously stated wishes."
- "Has the patient been given a chance to weigh in on this plan?"
- "I'm concerned that this approach may not align with our ethical responsibilities."

You don't have to have all the answers. You just have to be brave enough to ask the hard questions.

Moral Distress Is Real

Being ethically committed in an ethically complicated system can take a toll. Signs of **moral distress** include:

- Frustration with "the system"
- Emotional fatigue or helplessness
- Anger at repeated ethical compromises
- Questioning your career path

Talk about it. Journal. Seek peer support. Take breaks when you can. Ethics work is emotional labor—and it's okay to feel it.

Reflection Questions

- What ethical dilemma has stayed with you?
- How do you center your values when others want to move fast?
- Who do you turn to when you're navigating moral gray areas?

CHAPTER 14:
Health Equity and Social Justice

Not all patients arrive at the hospital with the same resources. Some have private insurance, stable housing, a family caregiver, and a network of support. Others arrive alone, uninsured, fearful, or carrying the weight of generational trauma and systemic injustice.

Health equity isn't just a buzzword—it's a moral imperative. As a medical social worker, **you are often the first to name the gap** between what is and what should be.

What Is Health Equity?

Health equity means that every person has a fair and just opportunity to be as healthy as possible—**regardless of race, gender, income, immigration status, language, disability, or location**.

It requires removing obstacles to care such as:

- Lack of insurance or access to providers
- Discrimination in healthcare settings
- Unsafe or unstable housing
- Food insecurity
- Transportation barriers
- Mistrust due to past harm or neglect

Equity doesn't mean giving everyone the same thing. It means giving people what they *need*.

What Health Inequity Looks Like in Practice

Scenario	Equity Lens
A patient delays care due to cost concerns	Offer charity care options or connect to financial assistance early
A patient with limited English receives minimal information	Ensure professional interpretation and health literacy support
A provider dismisses a patient's pain due to bias	Advocate for respectful, evidence-based care
A family lives in a food desert but needs a diabetic-friendly diet	Connect with local food access programs or case management
A patient without a phone misses follow-up appointments	Help access low-cost devices or community resources

These issues are not just inconvenient—they are **life-altering**. And they are everywhere.

Your Role as an Equity Advocate

Social workers don't just respond—we **interrupt** inequity by:

- Identifying barriers to care in real time
- Documenting social determinants of health in assessments
- Refusing to normalize biased or dismissive treatment
- Connecting patients to community-based supports
- Speaking up in team meetings when someone's needs are being overlooked

You might not be able to fix the system—but you can make it more humane for the person in front of you.

Build Your Equity Toolbox

To advocate effectively, know what's available in your area:

- Charity care applications
- Medication assistance programs
- Low-cost transportation options (e.g., Medicaid rides, rideshare partnerships)
- Clinics that serve uninsured or undocumented patients
- Mobile health units or home-visiting programs
- Community health workers or navigators

Build relationships with community partners who can do what the hospital can't.

Call Out, Call In

When you see inequity:

- **Call it out:** "I'm concerned that this discharge plan doesn't account for the patient's housing situation."
- **Call it in:** Bring others into the conversation, not to shame but to share responsibility: "Can we brainstorm together how to make this safer for them?"

Advocacy doesn't always mean conflict—it means courageous conversations.

Reflection Questions

- Where do you see the biggest gaps in care in your setting?
- How have you used your voice to advocate for a patient others overlooked?
- What resources or partnerships could help you expand your equity impact?

CHAPTER 15:
Understanding Healthcare Laws and Policies

Medical social workers walk a fine line—between advocacy and regulation, autonomy and protection, urgency and due process. To walk that line well, you must know the **rules of the system** you're working within.

You don't have to be a legal expert. However, you do need a working knowledge of the policies, laws, and ethical obligations that affect your patients and your role. When you understand the system, you're more empowered to help your patients *navigate* it—and when necessary, *challenge* it.

Key Laws Every Medical Social Worker Should Understand

Law/Policy	Why It Matters
HIPAA (Health Insurance Portability and Accountability Act)	Protects patient privacy and governs what information can be shared, with whom, and when
EMTALA (Emergency Medical Treatment and Labor Act)	Requires hospitals to screen and stabilize anyone who comes to the ER, regardless of insurance or ability to pay

Patient Self-Determination Act	Guarantees patients the right to make decisions about their care, including the right to refuse treatment
ADA (Americans with Disabilities Act)	Ensures equal access and prohibits discrimination based on disability
Mental Health Laws (vary by state)	Dictate involuntary holds, psychiatric evaluations, and patient rights in behavioral health settings
Mandated Reporting Laws	Define who must report abuse, what constitutes reportable harm, and how to document/report appropriately

Familiarity with these laws protects both your patients and your practice.

Why Policies and Procedures Matter

Every hospital or facility has internal policies. These:

- Clarify who can access records
- Define roles in discharge planning
- Outline steps for handling difficult patients
- Explain procedures for reporting ethical concerns

Read your policies. Keep them handy. Knowing them gives you the language and structure to advocate more effectively—and to protect yourself if your actions are questioned.

When Law and Ethics Clash

Sometimes, what the law allows and what your ethics demand don't align. For example:

- A patient's legal surrogate is making harmful decisions.
- You're asked to discharge a patient into an unsafe environment.
- Insurance denies coverage for essential services.

In these cases:

- Document everything clearly
- Consult ethics, legal, or risk management teams
- Use your Code of Ethics to guide advocacy
- Escalate concerns through appropriate channels

You may not be able to stop every injustice—but you can make sure your role reflects integrity and accountability.

Staying Current

Laws and policies change. To stay informed:

- Subscribe to your state's social work board or licensing body updates
- Attend continuing education focused on healthcare law
- Follow NASW, CMS, and local advocacy groups
- Build relationships with risk managers and compliance officers

What you know can shape what others *do*.

Reflection Questions

- What laws or policies do you refer to most often?
- Have you ever had to advocate using legal knowledge? What was the outcome?
- How do you stay informed about policy changes that affect your work?

Collaborative Practice

Medical social work doesn't happen in a vacuum. You work within complex systems—fast-moving hospitals, multi-disciplinary teams, community organizations—and your effectiveness depends on how well you can **collaborate** within those environments.

Section 4 is all about navigating **professional relationships**, systems of care, and the daily dance of teamwork in healthcare. You're not just there to speak for the patient—you're also there to connect dots, translate needs, and make things happen in real time.

This section will help you:

- Communicate clearly with physicians, nurses, and allied professionals
- Coordinate transitions across multiple care settings
- Write strong, defensible documentation that tells the full psychosocial story
- Organize resources and referrals in a way that supports outcomes
- Navigate conflict while centering the patient's voice

Your credibility as a social worker grows when you're seen as **reliable, responsive, and collaborative**—not just caring. This section will help you build that reputation while staying grounded in your ethics and expertise.

CHAPTER 16:
Communicating with Interdisciplinary Teams

No one works alone in a hospital or clinic. Patient care is a team effort—and medical social workers are essential team players. But to be effective in that role, you need to know how to communicate with diverse professionals: doctors, nurses, case managers, therapists, chaplains, and more.

Strong communication builds trust. It helps you advocate for patients, contribute to care planning, and earn your seat at the table.

Why Communication Matters

Interdisciplinary teams move fast. If your input isn't clear, timely, or aligned with the team's flow, it can get ignored or lost. But when you **communicate with clarity and clinical confidence**, your voice becomes one of the most valuable in the room.

Effective communication:

- Increases respect for the social work role
- Improves outcomes for patients and families
- Reduces misunderstandings and conflict
- Builds strong professional partnerships

Key Players on the Healthcare Team

Role	Focus
Physician/ APP	Diagnoses, treatment planning, and medical decision-making
Nurse	Day-to-day care, medication administration, patient monitoring
Case Manager	Insurance navigation, discharge coordination, length of stay
PT/OT/ST	Functional status, rehab potential, mobility, and communication
Pharmacist	Medication review and recommendations
Chaplain	Spiritual and emotional support
Social Worker	Psychosocial assessment, resource linkage, crisis support, advocacy

Each member sees a different side of the patient. Your goal is to **connect those perspectives** while representing the patient's story and needs.

The SBAR Technique for Clear Communication

A simple but effective format for team communication is **SBAR**:

- **S – Situation**: What's happening now?
- **B – Background**: What is the context?
- **A – Assessment**: What's your clinical judgment?
- **R – Recommendation**: What do you suggest or need from the team?

Example:

- *S – The patient is refusing discharge due to fear of going home alone.*
- *B – He lives in a third-floor walk-up, has no family support, and has fallen twice this year.*
- *A – He may need more supervision and support than initially thought.*
- *R – Can we explore a rehab placement while he regains strength?*

Tips for Being Heard by Medical Professionals

- **Speak their language.** Use clear, concise language with clinical relevance.
- **Time it right.** Ask to check in after rounds, not mid-crisis.
- **Be prepared.** Know the plan, prognosis, and discharge barriers before you speak up.
- **Stay solution-focused.** Don't just state the problem—offer a path forward.
- **Know when to escalate.** If concerns are dismissed, involve a supervisor or ethics consult.

Common Communication Pitfalls to Avoid

- Using jargon that isn't shared across disciplines
- Venting frustrations without a clear plan
- Over-explaining in high-pressure moments
- Withholding concerns because "they won't listen anyway"
- Speaking only from emotion rather than grounding in facts

Your Role as a Bridge

Social workers are **translators**—between systems, between disciplines, and between the medical team and the patient. You bring the human side of care into clinical conversations. That's not "soft"—it's essential.

Reflection Questions

- Who do you communicate with most often on the care team? What's working—and what's not?
- How do you ensure your voice is heard in interdisciplinary discussions?
- What communication habits could you strengthen to increase your effectiveness?

CHAPTER 17:
Coordinating Care Across Systems

Medical social work doesn't stop at the hospital door. Patients move across systems—hospital to rehab, rehab to home, home to outpatient, and sometimes back again. Each transition creates risk, and your role is to reduce that risk by ensuring **continuity of care**.

Coordinating care means connecting the dots—between providers, settings, insurance plans, and family members—so patients don't fall through the cracks.

Why Care Coordination Matters

Most readmissions happen within 30 days of discharge. Why? Because:

- Follow-up appointments are missed
- Prescriptions aren't filled
- Services aren't in place
- Families are overwhelmed
- There's no clear handoff

When care isn't coordinated, patients suffer. But when it is? Outcomes improve, satisfaction increases, and systems function better.

Systems You May Need to Coordinate With

System	Key Coordination Tasks
Post-Acute Care (SNF, IRF, LTAC)	Discharge planning, transfer notes, social summaries
Home Health/Hospice	Orders, equipment, caregiver education
Mental Health/ Substance Use	Referrals, crisis planning, safety supports
Primary Care/ Outpatient Clinics	Scheduling, record transfers, social history handoffs
Child/Adult Protective Services	Reports, follow-up contact, case coordination
Legal Systems	Guardianship, custody, court-mandated services
Housing/Shelter/ Community Services	Referral completion, eligibility documents, transportation

These systems often speak different "languages," operate on different timelines, and aren't always easy to reach. But patients rely on you to **make the handoff work**.

Essential Coordination Skills

- **Multitasking with intention:** Keep track of multiple moving parts without dropping details.
- **Follow-through:** A referral is only effective if someone receives it.
- **Relationship-building:** Know who to call and how to get a real answer.

- **Documentation:** Capture your coordination work clearly and professionally.
- **Patience + Persistence:** Sometimes, you have to follow up more than once—and that's okay.

The Warm Handoff

Whenever possible, create a **warm handoff**—a direct connection between you and the next provider:

- Speak by phone or in person
- Provide social context, not just clinical notes
- Include red flags, strengths, and recommendations
- Confirm the patient's understanding and involvement

A warm handoff builds trust between systems—and reduces "start-over" fatigue for patients.

Creating a Coordination Workflow

To stay organized:

- Use checklists or tracking sheets for referrals and follow-ups
- Color-code your tasks by urgency or discharge date
- Develop templates for common referrals
- Build a contact directory of reliable referral partners

Pro tip: A well-maintained spreadsheet can save you hours—and help during audits.

Reflection Questions

- What system transitions create the most stress for your patients?
- How do you track referrals and follow-ups?
- What tools or relationships help you coordinate care more effectively?

CHAPTER 18: Documentation that Matters

If it's not documented, it didn't happen.

Documentation is one of the most powerful tools in medical social work. It informs care, supports billing, protects against liability, and captures the psychosocial lens that others may overlook. Your notes are more than a paper trail—they're part of the patient's voice in the record.

Strong documentation reflects your professionalism, your clinical judgment, and your value to the team.

Why Documentation Matters

Clear, concise documentation:

- Ensures continuity of care
- Supports safe discharge planning
- Offers legal protection
- Demonstrates the need for social work services
- Helps colleagues understand psychosocial dynamics

When done well, your notes speak on your behalf long after you've left the room.

What to Document

Your documentation should answer:

1. **Why was social work involved?**
2. **What was the patient's situation or concern?**
3. **What action did you take?**
4. **What is the plan or outcome?**

Include:

- Psychosocial assessment findings
- Emotional responses and mental status
- Safety concerns
- Referrals made and coordination efforts
- Family or caregiver involvement
- Patient understanding and participation in the plan

Formats That Work

Common structures for social work documentation include:

SOAP Format:

- **S – Subjective** (What the patient or caregiver says)
- **O – Objective** (What you observe or gather factually)
- **A – Assessment** (Your clinical impression or concerns)
- **P – Plan** (What you did and next steps)

DAP Format:

- **D – Data** (Combined subjective/objective info)
- **A – Assessment** (Clinical interpretation)
- **P – Plan** (Actions, referrals, follow-up)

Use the format that aligns with your agency or EMR system—but **always write with intention and clarity**.

Tips for Strong Documentation

- **Be specific.** "Patient tearful and withdrawn" is stronger than "Patient upset."
- **Avoid assumptions.** Say "Patient reports," not "Patient is in denial."
- **Use quotes sparingly—but powerfully.** Especially when documenting exact wishes or distress.
- **Link to care.** Show how psychosocial issues impact treatment or discharge.
- **Document delays or barriers.** This is vital for accountability and advocacy.

What to Avoid

- Over-documenting things unrelated to care
- Using vague, judgmental, or coded language ("noncompliant" without explanation)
- Including personal opinions or irrelevant personal details
- Documenting outside your scope (diagnosing a medical or psychiatric condition)

Remember: patients have the right to access their records. Write with compassion and professionalism.

Your Documentation = Your Advocacy

Sometimes your note is the only place a patient's story gets recorded. A thoughtful psychosocial summary can shift a discharge decision, prompt a team meeting, or help a provider see the person behind the plan.

Reflection Questions

- What documentation habit do you want to strengthen?
- How do you balance being thorough with being efficient?
- How does your documentation reflect your voice, values, and clinical skills?

CHAPTER 19:
Leveraging Community Resources

One of the most visible and vital roles of a medical social worker is **resource navigation**. When patients need help beyond medical treatment—food, housing, transportation, mental health care, legal aid—they turn to you.

You are the connector. The lifeline. The person who knows *what's out there*, *how to get it*, and *what it takes* to qualify.

But here's the truth: systems are messy. Resources change. Eligibility rules shift. Programs open and close. The key is not just knowing resources—but knowing how to **work them**.

Types of Supportive Services Social Workers Often Refer To

Need	Examples of Resources
Housing	Transitional shelters, low-income housing programs, emergency motel vouchers, housing case managers
Food Security	Food banks, Meals on Wheels, SNAP applications, emergency grocery cards
Transportation	Medicaid rides, paratransit, rideshare partnerships, local volunteer driver programs

Medication Access	Prescription discount cards, manufacturer patient assistance programs, local pharmacy funding
Mental Health/ Substance Use	Outpatient therapy, detox programs, IOPs, crisis centers, support groups
Legal/Financial	Legal aid clinics, guardianship services, SSI/ SSDI support, utility assistance programs
Caregiving & Respite	Home health aides, adult day programs, caregiver support organizations

You won't always find the perfect match—but a **reasonable plan with a human touch** goes a long way.

How to Build Your Resource Toolbox

- **Keep a living document.** Update a digital resource guide quarterly.
- **Use folders or tags.** Organize resources by category, eligibility, and geography.
- **Vet your resources.** Have you called the number yourself? Visited the location? Ask patients about their experience.
- **Build relationships.** Get to know community liaisons. They're more likely to go the extra mile if they know you.
- **Don't reinvent the wheel.** Leverage lists from case managers, patient navigators, or discharge teams.

When Resources Are Scarce

You will face situations where there's **no easy solution**:

- No beds at the shelter
- No family to help

- No insurance coverage
- No time to wait on a waitlist

In those moments:

- Validate the frustration
- Offer what you *can* do
- Document all attempts
- Loop in supervisors or ethics if patient safety is at risk
- Stay connected and follow up when possible

Even a small win—a food bag, a bus pass, a call from someone who cares—can restore a patient's sense of hope.

Tips for Effective Referrals

- **Explain the why.** "This group helps people going through what you're experiencing."
- **Set realistic expectations.** "There may be a waitlist, but we can try together."
- **Involve the patient.** Don't just hand them a brochure—ask how they feel about it.
- **Confirm the connection.** When possible, call together, fax the referral, or email the contact directly.
- **Track your follow-up.** What did you send? When did they respond? Keep a record.

Reflection Questions

- What community resources do you rely on the most?
- How do you stay current with local services?
- What's one "creative" solution you've found for a complex social need?

CHAPTER 20:
Navigating Family and Team Conflicts

Where there are people, there will be conflict. In healthcare, where emotions run high and decisions carry weight, disagreements are inevitable. Whether it's a family fighting at the bedside or a care team clashing over treatment plans, **you** are often called in to make sense of the mess.

Conflict is not a failure—it's a signal. It means something important is at stake. Your job is not to take sides, but to help **everyone move forward with clarity, respect, and care**.

Common Conflict Scenarios in Medical Settings

- Family members disagree on end-of-life decisions
- A surrogate decision-maker makes choices that others question
- The care team and family have different goals (e.g., curative vs. comfort care)
- Patients feel unheard or disrespected by providers
- Providers are frustrated by a patient's choices or behaviors
- Cultural, spiritual, or communication differences cause tension

You won't always be able to resolve the conflict—but you can help hold space for resolution to *begin*.

What Conflict Really Needs

Conflict is often rooted in **fear, grief, guilt, powerlessness, or miscommunication**. Instead of trying to "fix" it, try to:

- Slow the moment down
- Identify the core issue underneath the disagreement
- Acknowledge emotions, even if they're messy
- Create space for everyone to feel heard
- Refocus on the patient's values and voice

You are a mirror, a translator, and a bridge—not a referee.

Facilitation Tips for Difficult Conversations

- **Set ground rules:** "Let's take turns speaking and try not to interrupt."
- **Use reflective listening:** "What I hear you saying is..."
- **Acknowledge emotion:** "This is incredibly hard. Everyone here cares deeply—that's part of why this feels so intense."
- **Redirect to the patient's wishes:** "What would your mother want if she were able to tell us right now?"
- **Clarify facts:** "Let's check with the physician so we're all on the same page medically."

Dealing with Team Conflict

Sometimes the conflict isn't between patient and family—it's *within the team*:

- A nurse and physician disagree on discharge readiness
- The team disagrees on patient capacity or next steps
- A provider dismisses your input or a patient's social barriers

In these moments:

- Stay calm and grounded in your role
- Use clinical language and clear documentation
- Ask clarifying questions rather than making accusations
- Involve a supervisor, ethics committee, or team huddle if needed

Your goal is to realign around the patient—not prove a point.

When Conflict Escalates

You are not responsible for fixing everything. But you **are** responsible for:

- Not escalating the situation further
- Not taking it personally
- Seeking support or backup when needed
- Documenting critical conversations and decisions
- Protecting your peace while showing up professionally

Sometimes, resolution takes time—and a return visit.

Reflection Questions

- What's a conflict you helped de-escalate recently? What worked?
- How do you stay centered when people are emotional or confrontational?
- What phrases or strategies help you lead with empathy in difficult conversations?

Growth and Leadership

Medical social work is demanding—mentally, emotionally, and physically. You carry stories of grief and resilience. You navigate broken systems, advocate for the unheard, and show up even when you're running on empty.

This final section is about *you*—your sustainability, your growth, and your impact beyond day-to-day tasks. Doing this work well means taking care of yourself while continuing to evolve as a professional.

In this section, you'll explore how to:

- Build a self-care practice that's realistic and restorative
- Understand licensure, supervision, and the path to leadership
- Embrace cultural humility as a lifelong process
- Lead through mentorship and example
- Stay current and connected in a rapidly changing healthcare landscape

Social work is a career—but it's also a calling. This section helps ensure that you don't just *do* the work—you stay well enough to *love* it for the long haul.

CHAPTER 21:
Building a Self-Care Practice

You can't pour from an empty cup—and in medical social work, your cup can empty fast. The emotional toll, ethical weight, and systemic barriers you navigate daily make this field both deeply meaningful and potentially exhausting.

Self-care isn't just about bubble baths and breathing exercises. It's about **sustainability**, boundaries, and creating systems that allow you to keep doing the work *without burning out.*

What Burnout Looks Like

Burnout doesn't always come with a breakdown. It sneaks in quietly:

- You dread your shift, even on your day off
- You feel detached or numb with patients
- You stop advocating because it "doesn't matter"
- Your documentation becomes mechanical
- You struggle to focus or feel emotionally drained after every interaction

Recognizing these signs early is key to protecting your well-being and professional integrity.

Types of Self-Care You Need

Domain	Examples
Physical	Sleep, hydration, stretching between cases, movement
Emotional	Journaling, therapy, processing with a trusted colleague
Professional	Regular supervision, realistic caseloads, clear boundaries
Spiritual	Mindfulness, nature, rituals, connecting to purpose
Relational	Spending time with people who see *you*, not just your role

Self-care is less about what you do and more about how often—and how intentionally—you do it.

Workplace Micro-Practices

You may not control your schedule, but you can create small pockets of care:

- Breathe intentionally between cases: 4 in, 4 hold, 4 out
- Step outside for two minutes of sunlight or silence
- Listen to music or a calming playlist during documentation
- Use a grounding object or sensory tool (stone, fidget, oil)

It's not self-indulgence—it's **emotional PPE**.

Setting and Holding Boundaries

Burnout often comes from saying yes to everything. Instead:

- Learn to say, "I can help with that after I complete this priority."
- Protect your breaks—yes, you *deserve* one
- Leave on time whenever possible
- Don't respond to work emails after hours unless it's part of your role

Boundaries are an act of integrity—not resistance.

The Role of Supervision and Peer Support

You don't need to process everything alone. Regular, high-quality supervision:

- Helps you reflect on emotional and ethical stressors
- Validates your experience
- Builds clinical skills and confidence

If you don't have formal supervision, consider:

- Forming a peer consult group
- Seeking mentorship from a seasoned colleague
- Requesting time during team meetings to debrief

Reflection Questions

- What are your early warning signs of burnout?
- What's one non-negotiable self-care practice you can commit to each week?
- How can you better advocate for your well-being in your work environment?

CHAPTER 22:
Licensure, Supervision, and Career Development

Social work isn't a static career—it's a journey of continuous learning and evolution. Whether you're fresh out of graduate school or a seasoned professional, understanding your **professional development path** is essential for both compliance and confidence.

In medical settings, licensure can determine your scope of practice, job eligibility, and advancement. Supervision helps you grow your clinical insight. Long-term growth ensures your career feels sustainable and meaningful—not just like a job.

Understanding Licensure

Licensing requirements vary by state, but typically include:

Credential	**Purpose**
LMSW (Licensed Master Social Worker)	Entry-level license; allows work under supervision
LCSW (Licensed Clinical Social Worker)	Independent practice, clinical assessment, psychotherapy
Advanced Clinical Licensure (state-specific)	May include board certification or specialty credentials

Make sure you know your state's:

- Required supervision hours
- Continuing education (CEU) requirements
- Renewal timelines
- Practice limitations under each license level

Pro tip: Keep a spreadsheet or digital folder to track hours, CEUs, and renewal dates.

Supervision That Supports Growth

Clinical supervision isn't just a box to check—it's where theory meets practice, and where you process what the textbooks never covered.

Effective supervision:

- Helps you navigate clinical dilemmas
- Supports ethical decision-making
- Offers space to process emotionally challenging cases
- Sharpens your interventions and assessments
- Encourages long-term career planning

Make the most of supervision by:

- Coming prepared with questions or cases
- Reflecting on emotional responses, not just logistics
- Seeking feedback regularly
- Asking to explore your *professional identity*, not just your paperwork

Career Growth Isn't Just About Climbing Ladders

There's no one path in social work. Growth might mean:

- Moving into leadership or program development
- Supervising students or early-career professionals
- Specializing in palliative care, transplant, or trauma

- Becoming an educator or policy advocate
- Opening a private practice

Don't just ask, "What's next?" Ask, **"What fits who I'm becoming?"**

Professional Development Tips

- Attend workshops and CEUs that truly interest you—not just the cheapest
- Join professional organizations (like NASW or specialty networks)
- Say yes to one thing a year that stretches your skill set
- Seek mentors who are doing the kind of work you admire
- Revisit your resume annually—even if you're not job-hunting

You don't have to grow fast. You just have to grow *intentionally*.

- ***Medical Social Worker Should Consider Getting CCM. Certified Case Manager (CCM)***
- ***Offered by the Commission for Case Manager Certification (CCMC)***
- ***Recognized across healthcare settings (hospitals, insurance, rehab)***
- ***Requires 12 months of case management experience and a healthcare license***

Reflection Questions

- Where are you in your licensure or supervision journey?
- What kind of support do you need to grow in your current role?
- What's one step you can take this month to invest in your professional future?

CHAPTER 23:
Practicing Cultural Humility

Cultural competence is not a destination—it's a lifelong practice. In healthcare, where power dynamics, access disparities, and historical harm intersect, **cultural humility** is not just recommended—it's *required.*

As a medical social worker, your patients will come from a wide range of backgrounds, identities, and lived experiences. They may not speak your language, hold your values, or trust the system you represent. That's why cultural humility is so important.

It allows you to offer care that is respectful, responsive, and grounded in the **reality of difference**—not just the theory of diversity.

What Is Cultural Humility?

Cultural humility is the practice of:

- Acknowledging that **you don't know everything**
- **Actively listening** to patients' experiences
- Recognizing **power imbalances** in healthcare relationships
- Being **open to feedback** and correction
- Committing to **lifelong learning**

Unlike cultural competence—which can suggest a "checklist" approach—humility asks you to **stay teachable**.

Why It Matters in Medical Social Work

You may work with:

- Immigrant or undocumented patients navigating fear and language barriers
- LGBTQ+ patients who've faced discrimination in healthcare settings
- Patients from historically marginalized racial or ethnic groups
- Families with spiritual beliefs that differ from medical norms
- Individuals with disabilities who are often spoken *about*, not *to*

In every case, cultural humility allows you to center the patient's identity and voice without making assumptions.

Culturally Humble Practice in Action

Situation	Cultural Humility Response
A patient declines a treatment due to religious beliefs	"Can you tell me more about how your beliefs guide your decisions?"
A patient prefers not to have male staff in the room	Respect the request and advocate for staffing that aligns
A family speaks a language you don't	Always use a professional interpreter—never rely on children or untrained staff
You make a mistake with a patient's name or pronoun	Apologize sincerely, correct yourself, and commit to doing better
You're unfamiliar with a cultural custom	Ask respectfully: "I'm not familiar with that tradition—would you be willing to share more with me?"

Bias Lives in All of Us

Cultural humility also means being willing to examine your own biases. Ask:

- Whose voices do I listen to most easily?
- What assumptions do I make based on appearance, accent, or age?
- How do my own experiences shape my lens—and where is that lens limited?

You are not "bad" for having bias. But you are responsible for what you do with it.

Build Your Cultural Awareness Toolkit

- Follow diverse voices in social work, medicine, and advocacy
- Attend trainings that stretch—not just confirm—your perspective
- Practice saying, "I don't know—can you help me understand?"
- Reflect on case experiences where culture played a central role
- Create space for feedback and dialogue within your team

Reflection Questions

- When have you been humbled by a patient's cultural perspective?
- How do you respond when you realize you've made a cultural misstep?
- What ongoing learning are you committed to in this area?

CHAPTER 24:
Mentorship and Teaching in the Medical Setting

You don't have to be a supervisor to be a leader. Some of the most impactful leadership in medical social work comes through quiet mentorship, modeling, and presence.

Whether you're guiding an intern, orienting a new hire, or simply being the person who stays calm during chaos, **you're teaching by how you work**.

Mentorship isn't about having all the answers—it's about making space for growth, reflection, and shared wisdom.

Why Mentorship Matters

Medical social work is demanding, and the learning curve is steep. Newer professionals often feel overwhelmed by the pace, the paperwork, and the emotional weight. A good mentor can:

- Normalize the stress and build resilience
- Offer practical tools and emotional support
- Model ethical practice and boundary setting
- Help someone find their professional identity
- Improve retention and team morale

You don't need a formal title to have this kind of impact.

Ways You Can Lead Right Now

Type of Leadership	What It Can Look Like
Mentorship	Offering to debrief after a tough case, reviewing notes, checking in
Field Instruction	Supervising MSW interns with intention and structure
Informal Teaching	Sharing tips, tools, or insights during team meetings
Advocacy Modeling	Speaking up respectfully when something isn't right
Supportive Presence	Holding space for overwhelmed teammates without judgment

Every conversation is an opportunity to lead with integrity and kindness.

Tips for Being an Effective Mentor or Teacher

- **Be honest, not harsh.** "Here's what worked well, and here's what I'd suggest next time."
- **Share your own mistakes.** It builds trust and reminds others they're not alone.
- **Stay open to learning.** Mentorship is a two-way street—your mentees will teach you, too.
- **Create psychological safety.** Make it okay to ask questions, struggle, or not know.
- **Encourage reflection.** "What felt most challenging in that interaction? What surprised you?"

What Makes a Lasting Impact

You don't have to be brilliant to be remembered—you just have to be present.

Often what mentees remember most is:

- The social worker who *noticed* they were struggling
- The one who *checked in* without an agenda
- The person who said, "You've got this," at just the right moment

Be that person.

Reflection Questions

- Who mentored you—and what did they teach you?
- What parts of your practice would you be proud to model for others?
- How can you create space for growth in your current role?

CHAPTER 25:
Staying Current in a Changing Field

Healthcare is not static. Policies shift, technologies evolve, patient needs change, and new research reshapes how we practice. If you want to remain effective and grounded, you have to stay curious, informed, and connected.

In a system that moves quickly and sometimes feels impersonal, **your relevance depends on your ability to grow**.

Why Staying Current Matters

When you stay up-to-date:

- You advocate with more confidence
- You bring new solutions to old challenges
- You prepare patients for what's next, not just what's now
- You protect your license, your reputation, and your clinical edge

And more importantly? You *don't burn out as easily*. Lifelong learning keeps your work fresh and connected to your sense of purpose.

What to Keep Up With

Topic	Why It Matters
Policy & Law Changes	Impacts patient rights, access, and your legal responsibilities

Insurance/Payor Shifts	Affects discharge planning, referrals, and patient financial stress
Medical Advances	Helps you understand new treatments, language, and care options
Social Work Best Practices	Keeps your interventions trauma-informed, ethical, and relevant
Cultural & Equity Trends	Ensures your care is inclusive, anti-oppressive, and responsive to real communities

You don't need to know everything—you just need to stay connected to what matters in your area of practice.

How to Stay Informed

- **Read one professional article a month.** Use journals like *Health & Social Work* or *Social Work in Health Care.*
- **Subscribe to newsletters.** Try NASW, state boards, hospital systems, or policy blogs.
- **Attend conferences, webinars, or CEUs** that stretch your thinking—not just meet requirements.
- **Join professional networks.** In-person or online groups help you share resources and support.
- **Talk to your peers.** Sometimes the best updates come from the colleague down the hall.

Your Growth = Your Impact

When you stay curious:

- You become a go-to person for your team
- You help others grow by sharing what you learn
- You shape the future of the profession—not just follow it

Remember, being "current" doesn't mean chasing every trend. It means being **awake to the world you work in**—and committed to showing up better each year than the last.

Reflection Questions

- What's one area of your practice you want to learn more about this year?
- How do you currently stay up-to-date—and what could you improve?
- Who inspires you to keep growing in this work?

Conclusion

Medical social work is more than just a profession; it's a calling. It requires resilience, adaptability, and a deep commitment to patient care. Mastering these 21 essential lessons equips you with the tools needed to navigate the complexities of healthcare, support your patients with confidence, and sustain a fulfilling career.

As you continue your journey, remember that learning never stops. The healthcare landscape is constantly evolving, and so should you. Stay curious, seek mentorship, and never hesitate to advocate for both your patients and yourself.

Most importantly, take care of yourself. The work you do is invaluable, but it can also be emotionally and physically demanding. Prioritizing your well-being isn't a luxury—it's a necessity.

Remember, know the power in your degree, and also when it is time to move on for the job.

Thank you for your dedication to this field. The impact you make, whether seen or unseen, is profound. Keep learning, keep growing, and keep making a difference.

Tools for Growth & Practice

Beyond clinical knowledge and compassionate care, thriving in medical social work requires access to real-world resources, professional insight, and lifelong learning tools. This bonus section equips you with practical materials to support your daily work, deepen your understanding, and expand your career possibilities.

You'll explore:

- Case Studies – Real-world scenarios with clinical reflection and analysis
- Glossary of Terms – Common healthcare and social work terminology at your fingertips
- Recommended Reading – Books and resources to sharpen your skills and perspective
- Professional Organizations & Conferences – Where to connect, learn, and lead in the field
- Sample Job Descriptions – Insight into roles and expectations across diverse settings

This final section offers a springboard for continued growth, professional networking, and real-life application—so you can keep evolving as a confident, competent medical social worker.

CASE STUDY 1:
The Unsafe Discharge

Chapter Tie-In: *Chapter 9 – Discharge Planning*

Setting: Inpatient Hospital – General Medicine

Background: Mr. R, a 63-year-old man with poorly controlled diabetes, was admitted for a foot infection that required partial amputation. He is being discharged after a 9-day stay. He uses a wheelchair, has no phone, lives on the third floor of an apartment with no elevator, and has no family support. His Medicaid transportation expired.

Social Work Challenge: The team plans to discharge him with home health, but you recognize the home environment is not accessible or safe. The attending says, "There's nothing more we can do—we need the bed."

Reflection Questions:

1. What immediate safety risks are present if the discharge proceeds?
2. What systems or supports could you advocate for in this situation?
3. How would you document this ethically and clinically?

Analysis: This situation requires strong advocacy. Call a care conference. Propose SNF placement or short-term rehab if eligible. Document barriers, communicate with risk management, and, if needed, involve adult protective services. Ethically, your role is to protect the patient's dignity and safety—not just flow with the discharge timeline.

CASE STUDY 2:
The Capacity Conflict

Chapter Tie-In: *Chapter 11 – Autonomy & Consent*

Setting: Emergency Department

Background: Ms. L, a 72-year-old with dementia, presents with a UTI and signs of confusion. Her daughter insists on signing surgical consent for a procedure that Ms. L had previously refused when she was alert. The ED staff wants to proceed.

Social Work Challenge: You question whether the daughter is overriding the patient's known wishes and whether true consent has been obtained.

Reflection Questions:

1. What steps must be taken to assess capacity before a surrogate can decide?
2. How would you advocate for a pause in this situation?
3. Who else should be looped in?

Analysis: You can ask for a formal capacity evaluation. Present Ms. L's previously stated wishes and document clearly. Collaborate with the ethics committee or legal team if the daughter is acting outside the scope of her power. You are advocating for Ms. L's autonomy, even in altered states.

CASE STUDY 3:
The Family Rift at End-of-Life

Chapter Tie-In: *Chapter 7 – Supporting Loss and End-of-Life*

Setting: ICU

Background: A patient is intubated with no chance of recovery. His wife wants to withdraw life support and follow the patient's wishes. His adult children (from a previous marriage) arrive and demand continued treatment, yelling at staff and threatening to sue.

Social Work Challenge: You're asked to mediate the conflict while keeping the unit calm and ensuring the patient's wishes are respected.

Reflection Questions:

1. How do you balance the legal decision-maker's rights with family distress?
2. How would you structure a family meeting in this emotionally charged situation?
3. What tools help you de-escalate tension?

Analysis: Facilitate a structured meeting with medical, palliative, and chaplain support. Center the patient's values. Acknowledge grief as the root of conflict, and clarify the wife's legal role. Document all conversations and provide grief support resources. Sometimes, naming the pain helps resolve the fight.

CASE STUDY 4:
No Place to Go

Chapter Tie-In: *Chapter 14 – Health Equity and Access*

Setting: Urban Hospital

Background: Mr. T is a 50-year-old unhoused man with HIV and schizophrenia. He's medically stable but has nowhere to go after discharge. He needs meds, food, and psychiatric follow-up but refuses a shelter due to past trauma. The hospital can't keep him, and outpatient services are waitlisted.

Social Work Challenge: You're told to "just find a place" and discharge him today.

Reflection Questions:

1. What equity issues are present in this situation?
2. How do you balance patient autonomy with system limitations?
3. What does trauma-informed advocacy look like here?

Analysis: This case highlights systemic failure. Explore warming centers, street outreach teams, or harm-reduction drop-in sites. Involve the patient in every decision. Document his preferences, the barriers, and all attempted referrals. Loop in a community-based social worker or mobile crisis if possible.

CASE STUDY 5:
The First-Year Social Worker

Chapter Tie-In: *Chapter 21 – Self-Care*

Setting: Large Trauma Hospital – Behavioral Health Unit

Background: You're an LMSW 3 months into your job. After a string of deaths, aggressive family encounters, and high caseloads, you find yourself crying in the breakroom and dreading every shift. You feel guilty taking time off and worry you're not "cut out" for the field.

Social Work Challenge: You need to advocate for your well-being—but aren't sure how.

Reflection Questions:

1. What are the signs that you may be approaching burnout?
2. Who can you talk to in your workplace for support?
3. What does realistic self-care look like in your setting?

Analysis: This is a time for reflection and re-grounding. Seek supervision, consider short-term therapy, and request support from your manager or EAP. Take intentional breaks. You're not failing—you're learning to sustain. Build peer connections and revisit your "why." You *do* belong here.

Glossary of Terms for Medical Social Workers

A – D

- **Advance Directive** – A legal document outlining a person's wishes for medical care if they become unable to speak for themselves.
- **APS (Adult Protective Services)** – State agency that investigates reports of abuse, neglect, or exploitation of vulnerable adults.
- **Capacity** – A clinical determination of whether a patient can understand, evaluate, and communicate decisions about their care.
- **Case Management** – Coordinated services that help individuals meet health and social service needs through planning, referrals, and advocacy.
- **Charting/Documentation** – The written record of care provided, used for communication, legal, and billing purposes.
- **Cognitive Impairment** – A reduction in mental functions such as memory, problem-solving, or attention, which may affect decision-making.
- **Consent (Informed)** – Voluntary agreement to treatment or services based on a clear understanding of risks, benefits, and alternatives.
- **COPD (Chronic Obstructive Pulmonary Disease)** – A progressive lung disease that makes breathing difficult.

D – H

- **Discharge Planning** – The process of preparing a patient to leave a medical facility and ensuring a safe, supported transition.
- **DME (Durable Medical Equipment)** – Medically necessary equipment (e.g., walkers, oxygen, hospital beds) provided for home use.
- **ED (Emergency Department)** – The hospital department that provides immediate care for urgent or life-threatening conditions.
- **Ethics Committee** – A multidisciplinary group that consults on complex healthcare decisions involving ethical dilemmas.
- **Family Meeting** – A structured conversation with patients, family members, and care team members to discuss care goals and plans.
- **Full Code / DNR (Do Not Resuscitate)** – Indicates whether or not a patient wants CPR or life-saving interventions in a medical emergency.

H – P

- **HIPAA (Health Insurance Portability and Accountability Act)** – U.S. law that protects the privacy and security of health information.
- **Home Health** – Medical or supportive services provided in a patient's home under physician orders.
- **Hospice** – Specialized care for individuals with a terminal illness, focused on comfort, dignity, and quality of life.
- **ICU (Intensive Care Unit)** – A hospital unit that provides intensive monitoring and treatment for critically ill patients.
- **Interdisciplinary Team (IDT)** – A group of professionals (doctors, nurses, social workers, etc.) collaborating to deliver holistic care.
- **Mandatory Reporter** – A professional required by law to report suspected abuse, neglect, or exploitation.

- **MPOA (Medical Power of Attorney)** – A legal document that designates someone to make healthcare decisions on behalf of a patient.
- **Multidisciplinary Rounds** – Daily or regular team discussions about patient care planning and progress.

P – Z

- **Palliative Care** – Specialized medical care for people with serious illness, focused on symptom relief and quality of life.
- **POLST/MOST** – Physician/Medical Orders for Life-Sustaining Treatment, specific medical orders based on a patient's care preferences.
- **Post-Acute Care** – Services that help patients recover after hospitalization, such as rehab, skilled nursing, or home care.
- **Protective Hold (Involuntary Hold)** – A legal intervention used when a patient poses a risk to self or others due to mental health crisis.
- **Psychosocial Assessment** – A clinical evaluation of a patient's emotional, social, spiritual, and environmental factors.
- **SNF (Skilled Nursing Facility)** – A licensed facility that provides short-term rehab or long-term nursing care.
- **Social Determinants of Health (SDOH)** – Conditions in which people live, work, and grow that influence health outcomes.
- **Trauma-Informed Care** – An approach that acknowledges the prevalence and impact of trauma and seeks to avoid re-traumatization.

Recommended Reading for Medical Social Workers

Medical Social Work & Healthcare Systems

- **"Social Work Practice in Health Care"** by Karen M. Allen
- *A comprehensive guide to roles, settings, and skills specific to social workers in medical environments.*
- **"Medical Social Work: Evidence-Based Practice"** by Ruth E. Chenitz & Jill Black
- *Focuses on research-informed strategies in hospital and outpatient settings.*
- **"From Silence to Voice: What Nurses Know and Must Communicate to the Public"** by Bernice Buresh & Suzanne Gordon
- *Though written for nurses, this book offers insight into interprofessional dynamics and patient advocacy.*
- **"Crucial Conversations: Tools for Talking When Stakes Are High"** by Patterson, Grenny, McMillan, and Switzler
- *Useful for family meetings, difficult discharges, and advocacy within interdisciplinary teams.*
- **"Motivational Interviewing in Health Care"** by Stephen Rollnick, William R. Miller, and Christopher Butler
- *A practical guide for using MI techniques to support behavior change and engagement in healthcare settings.*
- **"Narrative Medicine: Honoring the Stories of Illness"** by Rita Charon
- *Encourages clinicians to deeply engage with patient narratives as part of healing and care planning.*

Professional Organizations & Conferences for Medical Social Workers

National Professional Organizations

- **National Association of Social Workers (NASW)**

  www.socialworkers.org

  The leading voice for social work in the U.S., offering advocacy, licensing guidance, professional development, ethics resources, and state chapters.

  ➤ *Annual NASW Conference* (National + State Chapters)

- **Society for Social Work Leadership in Health Care (SSWLHC)**

  www.sswlhc.org

  Focused specifically on healthcare social work leadership, ethics, and policy.

  ➤ *Annual Meeting and Conference*

- **Council on Social Work Education (CSWE)**

  www.cswe.org

  Governs social work education standards and supports continuing education and accreditation.

  ➤ *Annual Program Meeting (APM)*

- **National Hospice and Palliative Care Organization (NHPCO)** www.nhpco.org

Resources and training for social workers in end-of-life and palliative care.

➤ *Interdisciplinary Conference (IDEC)*

- **American Case Management Association (ACMA)**

  www.acmaweb.org

  Offers resources and certification for case management professionals across healthcare settings.

  ➤ *National and State Conferences*

Specialty & Intersectional Organizations

- **Clinical Social Work Association (CSWA)**

  www.clinicalsocialworkassociation.org

  Advocates for clinical practice rights, standards, and reimbursement.

- **National Association of Black Social Workers (NABSW)**

  www.nabsw.org

  Supports African American social workers and the communities they serve.

- **Latino Social Workers Organization (LSWO)**

  www.lswo.org

  Promotes culturally informed practice and networking for Latinx social workers.

- **International Federation of Social Workers (IFSW)**

www.ifsw.org

Global voice of the profession—resources, ethics, and international conference opportunities.

- **Society for Spirituality & Social Work**

  www.spiritualityandsocialwork.org

  Explores the integration of spiritual care into social work practice—valuable for medical and hospice settings.

Conferences to Watch

Conference	Focus
NASW National Conference	Policy, ethics, supervision, direct practice
SSWLHC Annual Conference	Healthcare systems, leadership, clinical topics
NHPCO Interdisciplinary Conference	End-of-life care, grief, hospice social work
ACMA National Conference	Case management, transitions of care, utilization review
CSWE APM	Education, research, field training, and social work curriculum innovation
State NASW Conferences	Region-specific networking, CEUs, advocacy work

Sample Job Descriptions

1. Medical Social Worker – Inpatient Hospital (General Medicine)

Setting: Urban Acute Care Hospital

Schedule: Full-Time | Monday–Friday with occasional weekends

Key Responsibilities:

- Conduct psychosocial assessments and discharge planning
- Provide support to patients and families during hospitalization
- Coordinate post-acute referrals (SNFs, rehab, home health)
- Respond to crises (e.g., abuse, grief, mental health)
- Collaborate with physicians, nurses, and case managers
- Document services in the EMR in compliance with hospital policy

Qualifications:

- MSW required; LMSW or LCSW preferred
- 1–2 years of medical social work experience
- Knowledge of Medicaid/Medicare, DME, and community resources
- Strong communication, assessment, and problem-solving skills

2. Palliative Care Social Worker – Outpatient Oncology Clinic

Setting: Cancer Center / Palliative Care Program

Schedule: Full-Time | Flexible Day Hours

Key Responsibilities:

- Provide counseling, emotional support, and resource navigation
- Facilitate advance care planning and support goals-of-care conversations
- Educate patients and families about hospice and comfort care options
- Collaborate with palliative physicians, nurses, and chaplains
- Assess caregiver needs and link to respite and mental health services

Qualifications:

- MSW required; LCSW and ACHP-SW certification preferred
- Minimum 2 years of experience in hospice or palliative care
- Training in grief and loss, trauma-informed care, and communication
- Deep empathy, calm presence, and ethical clarity required

3. Behavioral Health Social Worker – Emergency Department

Setting: Level I Trauma Center Emergency Department

Schedule: 12-Hour Shifts | Nights, Weekends, and Holidays

Key Responsibilities:

- Complete behavioral health and suicide risk assessments
- Initiate psychiatric holds when indicated per state law

- Coordinate inpatient psych placements and community follow-up
- Collaborate with security, police, psych staff, and nursing team
- Provide brief intervention and de-escalation

Qualifications:

- MSW required; LCSW or LMSW with supervised experience
- At least 1 year in behavioral health or ER setting
- Familiarity with local psychiatric facilities and legal hold process
- Strong crisis management and documentation skills

4. Home Health & Hospice Social Worker

Setting: Community-Based | Patient Homes & Facilities

Schedule: Full-Time | Travel Required

Key Responsibilities:

- Conduct psychosocial assessments in. the home environment
- Address barriers to care: housing, food, caregiver burnout
- Support end-of-life planning and family grief processes
- Link patients to in-home supportive services and benefits
- Coordinate with nurses, aides, spiritual care, and volunteers

Qualifications:

- MSW required; LCSW preferred
- Minimum 1 year of experience in hospice, home care, or geriatrics
- Comfortable working independently in patients' homes
- Knowledge of Medicare hospice benefit, ethics, and cultural sensitivity

5. Social Work Case Manager – Managed Care Organization

Setting: Health Plan/Insurance Company (Remote or Hybrid)

Schedule: Monday–Friday | Business Hours

Key Responsibilities:

- Conduct telephonic case management with high-risk members
- Authorize services, coordinate transitions of care, and monitor outcomes
- Assist members with health literacy, access barriers, and benefit use
- Maintain documentation for audits and utilization review
- Serve as liaison between providers, members, and families

Qualifications:

- MSW required; LCSW or certification in case management (CCM or C-ASWCM) preferred
- 2+ years in healthcare navigation or insurance setting
- Strong technology, communication, and organization skills
- Knowledge of population health, Medicaid/Medicare, and managed care models

About the Author

Dr. Kenshara Cravens-Knoxson believes everyone is capable of change. It's this tenet that led to pursuing her calling in Social Work. With a singular goal of empowering many, she finds ways to contribute through service, mentorship, and compassion.

A first-generation college student, Dr. Cravens-Knoxson understands the value of knowledge and the struggle involved in overcoming diversities. As such, she continuously seeks opportunities to expand and develop her education.

Dr. Cravens-Knoxson earned her Ph.D. in Social Work from Walden University in 2023. Her dissertation is titled, "Experiences and Perceptions of Hospital Social Workers," wherein she explores the commonly misunderstood world of social work in hospitals. A subject she knows well as she'll also be earning the title of Licensed Clinical Social Worker (LCSW) this year.

She is a Licensed Master Social Worker (LMSW) and a Licensed Graduate Social Worker (LGSW) and serves as an Assistant Professor at Prairie View A&M University. As Assistant Professor, Dr. Cravens-Knoxson runs an active and dynamic classroom, keeping students engaged with community-building exercises as part of the curriculum. She conducts numerous lectures and seminars with panache.

While it's no secret that Dr. Cravens-Knoxson is an unstoppable force, there are a few accomplishments she holds close to her heart: The

Sages of Clinical Services Award 2021, presented by United Healthcare. Bestowed to a handful of worthy recipients from a pool of over 50,000, the award is given to licensed clinicians who continually embody United Health values, including ethics, sympathy, and the fostering of relationships.

Dr. Cravens-Knoxson made the "40 Under 40" list presented by the Galveston Daily News. Recognized for being a young professional devoted to personal and professional growth, and for her commitment to the community.

She received the Hometown Hero Award, presented by *The Carolyn Taylor Lee* Foundation. The Non-Profit organization has a goal of providing daily support to communities throughout the year, empowering households with a family-centric unit in mind.

Inspired by her achievements in the Non-Profit space, Dr. Cravens-Knoxson established *Craving for A Change Foundation, Inc.* The foundation's overarching goal is to institute social-emotional learning strategies for adolescent and young adult students attending the Galveston County public school system.

With social work and youth ever present as her impetus, Dr. Cravens-Knoxson is a maven in her field. As she continues to fuel her appetite for knowledge and works to empower her peers, she looks forward to what the future holds.

Made in the USA
Monee, IL
04 November 2026

67383012R00066